POCKET GUIDES

CW00486442

LEARNING DISABILITY PLACEMENTS

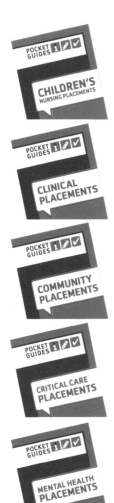

Pocket Guides

A unique series of pocket-sized books designed to help nursing and healthcare students make the most of their practice learning experiences.

"All the information was clear and concise, this book is exactly what I was looking for." ★★★★★

"A great little guide. All the basic information needed to have a quick reference." ★★★★★

"A very useful, well-written and practical pocket book for any level of student nurse preparing for placement." ★★★★★

"Written by students for students. A must for any student about to head on placement." ★★★★★

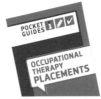

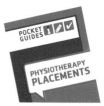

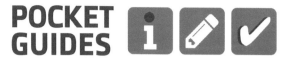

POCKET GUIDES

LEARNING DISABILITY PLACEMENTS

Edited by Sam Humphrey

De Montfort University, Leicester

Lantern

ISBN: 9781908625892
First published in 2021 by Lantern Publishing Ltd

Lantern Publishing Limited, The Old Hayloft, Vantage
Business Park, Bloxham Road, Banbury OX16 9UX, UK
www.lanternpublishing.com

© 2021, Justine Barksby, Adele Bunten, Kathleen Dabbs, Patrick
Hugh Doherty, Helen Doughty, Mark Ellis, Hannah Greenwood,
Sam Humphrey, Jemma Lockwood, Adele Postance and Richard
Postance. The right of Justine Barksby, Adele Bunten, Kathleen
Dabbs, Patrick Hugh Doherty, Helen Doughty, Mark Ellis, Hannah
Greenwood, Sam Humphrey, Jemma Lockwood, Adele Postance
and Richard Postance to be identified as authors of this work has
been asserted by them in accordance with the Copyright, Designs
and Patents Act 1988.

All rights reserved. No part of this publication may be reproduced,
stored in a retrieval system, copied or transmitted in any form or
by any means, electronic, mechanical, photocopying, recording
or otherwise without either written permission from Lantern
Publishing Ltd or by a licence permitting restricted copying in the
UK issued by the Copyright Licensing Agency, Saffron House, 6–10
Kirby Street, London EC1N 8TS, UK.
www.cla.co.uk

British Library Cataloguing in Publication Data
A catalogue record for this book is available from the British Library

The authors and publisher have made every attempt to ensure
the content of this book is up to date and accurate. However,
healthcare knowledge and information is changing all the time
so the reader is advised to double-check any information in
this text on drug usage, treatment procedures, the use of
equipment, etc. to confirm that it complies with the latest safety
recommendations, standards of practice and legislation, as well as
local Trust policies and procedures. Students are advised to check
with their tutor and/or practice supervisor before carrying out
any of the procedures in this textbook.

Typeset by Medlar Publishing Solutions Pvt Ltd, India
Printed and bound in the UK

Last digit is the print number: 10 9 8 7 6 5 4 3 2 1

Personal information

Name:..

Mobile:..

Address during placement:...........................

UNIVERSITY DETAILS

University: ....

Programme leader: ....

Personal tutor:....................................

PLACEMENT DETAILS

Placement area:....................................

Practice Education Facilitator:.....................

Link lecturer: ....

CONTACT IN CASE OF EMERGENCY

Name:..

Contact number (mobile):............................

Contact number (home/work):.........................

Contents

Preface

This pocket guide to learning disability nursing placements has been specifically written for student learning disability nurses. It acknowledges that the field of learning disability nursing is a unique and specialist profession and that student learning disability nurses will need an arsenal of distinctive knowledge and skills at their disposal.

Within learning disability services, you will find a variety of abbreviations and terms used to refer to learning disabilities and people with learning disabilities, such as patients or service users. For the purposes of this guide, we have used the abbreviation 'LD' for learning disability/disabilities and 'person' wherever possible as a reminder that a person with learning disabilities should not be defined by their diagnostic label.

Sam Humphrey

Lecturer in Learning Disability Nursing
De Montfort University, Leicester

List of contributors

Dr Justine Barksby
Senior Lecturer in Learning Disability Nursing, The Leicester School of Nursing and Midwifery, De Montfort University, Leicester

- *Sections contributed to: 6.2, 12.3, 13.4, 13.5, 13.9 and 18*

Adele Bunten
Student Learning Disability Nurse, The Leicester School of Nursing and Midwifery, De Montfort University, Leicester

- *Sections contributed to: 13.1, 13.7, 13.10, 20 and 21*

Kathleen Dabbs
Senior Lecturer in Learning Disability and Children's Nursing, The Leicester School of Nursing and Midwifery, De Montfort University, Leicester

- *Section contributed to: 13.12*

Patrick Hugh Doherty
Student Learning Disability Nurse, The Leicester School of Nursing and Midwifery, De Montfort University, Leicester

- *Sections contributed to: 15.1, 15.2 and 21*

Helen Doughty
Lecturer in Children's Nursing, The Leicester School of Nursing and Midwifery, De Montfort University, Leicester

- *Section contributed to: 12.2*

Mark Ellis
Senior Lecturer in Mental Health Nursing, The Leicester School of Nursing and Midwifery, De Montfort University, Leicester

- *Sections contributed to: 6.1 and 13.6*

Hannah Greenwood
Learning Disability Primary Care Liaison Nurse,
Nottinghamshire Healthcare NHS Foundation Trust

- *Section contributed to: 15.4*

Sam Humphrey
Lecturer in Learning Disability Nursing, The Leicester School
of Nursing and Midwifery, De Montfort University, Leicester

- *Sections contributed to: 4, 5, 10, 12.1, 12.2, 13.1, 13.3, 13.7,
  13.10, 15.3, 16, 17, 19, 20 and 21*

Jemma Lockwood
Practice Lead, The Leicester School of Nursing and Midwifery,
De Montfort University, Leicester

- *Sections contributed to: 2, 3, 7, 8 and 9*

Adele Postance
Admissions Nurse, Rainbows Hospice for Children and Young
People, Leicestershire

- *Section contributed to: 13.8*

Richard Postance
Senior Lecturer in Learning Disability Nursing, The Leicester
School of Nursing and Midwifery, De Montfort University,
Leicester

- *Sections contributed to: 6.3, 11, 13.2, 13.11 and 14*

Acknowledgements

We would like to thank the LD student nurses in cohorts 1703, 1709, 1809 and 1909 from the Leicester School of Nursing and Midwifery at De Montfort University, Leicester for their contributions in developing content and sharing their experiences.

We would also like to thank the authors of the other Pocket Guide books in the series for the inspiration they gave us from their sections and content.

Abbreviations

Abbreviations can vary between clinical areas and can mean different things to different people in different contexts, so always check.

Abbreviations common in LD services

AAC	augmentative and alternative communication
ADHD	attention deficit hyperactivity disorder
ADL	activities of daily living
ASD	autistic spectrum disorder
ATU	assessment and treatment unit
CAMHS	child and adolescent mental health services
CLDN	community learning disability nurse
CLDT	community learning disability team
DoLS	Deprivation of Liberty Safeguards
HAP	health action plan
LD/ID	learning disability/intellectual disability
LeDeR	Learning Disabilities Mortality Review programme
LPS	liberty protection safeguards
MCA	Mental Capacity Act
PBS	positive behaviour support
PCC	person-centred care
PECS	Picture Exchange Communication System
PEG	percutaneous endoscopic gastrostomy
PEJ	percutaneous endoscopic jejunostomy
PMLD	profound and multiple learning disabilities
RNLD	registered nurse learning disabilities
STOMP	stopping over-medication of people with a learning disability, autism or both
VNS	vagus nerve stimulator

Abbreviations common in general services

A&E	Accident and Emergency
ABC	airway, breathing, circulation
ANTT	aseptic non-touch technique
A(D)PIE	assessment, (diagnosis), planning, implementation, evaluation
BLS	Basic Life Support
BNO	bowels not opened
BO	bowels opened
BP	blood pressure
CBT	cognitive behavioural therapy
CD	controlled drug
CPA	care programme approach
CPR	cardiopulmonary resuscitation
DHSC	Department of Health and Social Care
DNR/DNAR/DNACPR	do not attempt resuscitation
DOB	date of birth
DOH	Department of Health
GP	general practitioner
ICD	International Classification of Diseases
IM	intramuscular
IOF	incontinent of faeces
IOU	incontinent of urine
IV	intravenous
MAR	medication administration record
MDT	multidisciplinary team
MHA	Mental Health Act
NAD	no abnormality detected
NAI	non-accidental injury

NBM	nil by mouth
NG	nasogastric
NJ	nasojejunal
NMC	Nursing and Midwifery Council
O_2	oxygen
OCD	obsessive–compulsive disorder
PD	personality disorder
PHE	Public Health England
PO	taken orally
PR	given rectally
PRN	give as required
PU	passed urine
RR	respiratory rate
SC	subcutaneous
TPN	total parenteral nutrition
TPR	temperature, pulse, respirations
UTI	urinary tract infection

The 6 Cs of nursing values

Care

Compassion

Courage

Communication

Commitment

Competence

Before we start

Placement

- Every placement provides learning opportunities; make the most of every one.
- Research common LD conditions, as you will encounter these most often.
- Understand common medications for people with LD.
- Remember that it's OK to be sick. We don't want to pass on anything to people with LD, who may be more susceptible to illnesses. Be sure to let placement and university know if you're unwell.

University and placement

- Use a reflective cycle that works for you; pick one that you like and find easy to use.
- Ask for support if you need it. Whether at university or on placement your personal tutor, academic assessor, practice assessor and practice supervisor are your support mechanism – use them.

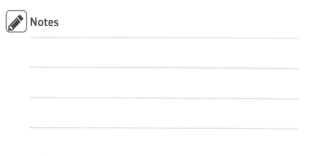 Notes

Getting there

Top tips

Take time to prepare for placement; this will help you to settle in quickly. Some useful preparatory suggestions are:

- Arrange a pre-placement visit.
- Find out the date and time of your first few shifts.
- Plan your travel – consider doing a practice run. If you're driving, ask about parking arrangements ahead of time; if you're on public transport, check your travel times will fit your shifts.
- Ask for the placement induction pack – these will often contain a wealth of useful placement-specific information.
- Find out about the uniform policy. If a placement area does not require you to wear uniform, smart clothing will still be required; be guided by the local policy of the placement area. Pockets can be useful to carry pens, etc. Try not to take valuables with you to placement, as not all placements have lockers available for students.
- Research the clinical specialism of your placement area.
- Find out the arrangements for food/lunch. Some placement areas will provide meals for a small charge, others may have on-site canteens or local shops/facilities available nearby. If you have a community placement you may need to bring your own drinks as well as food.
- Remember to bring this pocket guide!

✔ Record tasks you may like to add:

☐ _____

☐ _____

☐ _____

☐ _____

☐ _____

☐ _____

☐ _____

☐ _____

☐ _____

☐ _____

☐ _____

☐ _____

5

You will need to inform your placement area at the earliest opportunity if you're unable to attend as scheduled for any reason. Find out from your Practice Supervisor who you will need to contact and make a note of their details below.

Name:

Contact:

Remember to follow both the placement and university policy with regard to reporting absence. This will detail who to contact and when, as well as how often you need to keep in touch during your absence.

When you're ready to return to placement contact your Practice Supervisor to negotiate this, and remember to keep your university informed. If you feel you need reasonable adjustments to facilitate your return, discuss this with your practice supervisor in the first instance. Your practice supervisor will update your timesheet on your return. Follow local/university policy with regard to retrieving hours.

The NMC Code

The Nursing and Midwifery Council (NMC) is the professional regulating body for nurses in the UK. It provides a code of professional standards of practice and behaviour that all registered nurses, midwives and nursing associates must follow. The Code is grouped into four key themes and these are summarised below.

> Read the Code at **bit.ly/NMC-Code**
>
> To make it easy for you to access them, we have shortened web links to this format – simply type these into any web browser and you'll go to the right page!

Prioritise people

- Treat people as individuals and uphold their dignity
- Listen to people and respond to their preferences and concerns
- Make sure that people's physical, social and psychological needs are assessed and responded to
- Always act in the best interests of people
- Respect people's right to privacy and confidentiality

Practise effectively

- Always practise in line with evidence
- Communicate clearly   *see Section 11*
- Work cooperatively and share your skills, knowledge and experience
- Keep clear and accurate records – make sure another registered nurse reads and countersigns your documentation
- Be accountable for your decisions

Preserve safety

- Recognise and work within the limits of your competence – speak to your practice supervisor if you're asked to do something you're not confident about
- Be open and honest – especially if you make a mistake
- Always offer help in an emergency
  - make sure you know how to call for emergency help in your placement area
- Know how to raise concerns if you believe someone's safety is at risk see *Section 6.3*

Promote professionalism and trust

- Always uphold the reputation of your profession
  - this includes when you're studying at university and in your personal life
  - your social media posts are also included in this 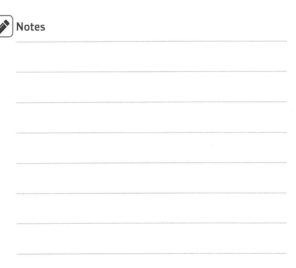 see *Section 7*

📝 Notes

Person-centred care

Person-centred care (PCC) is about always putting the person you're supporting at the centre of your decision making and considering how you can promote their independence and meet their unique circumstances.

A framework specific to LD practice has been developed to support the LD nursing focus on PCC, evidence-based practice and reflection. The application of the Moulster and Griffiths LD nursing model (see inside front cover) is based partly on the APIE nursing process (assess, plan, implement and evaluate). This model expands the APIE approach to consider PCC with people with LD.

See *Sections 13.1* and *13.2* for more on assessment and care planning

Nursing process	Moulster and Griffiths model
Assessment	1. Person-centred screen
	2. Nursing assessment
	3. Health Equality Framework baseline — see *Section 13.1*
Planning	4. Nursing care plan
Implementation	5. Nursing implementation
Evaluation	6. Health Equality Framework
	7. Care plan evaluation

For more about the Moulster and Griffiths model see bit.ly/MG-LD

Related to PCC, 'diagnostic overshadowing' is making decisions based upon diagnostic labels that we attach to

9

people, and making assumptions about them because of these labels. The result of this is that it risks losing sight of the individual person and how they might go about expressing their individual needs. As LD nurses, person-centred care should always be at the heart of what we do and how we practise.

Top tips

- Always put the person with LD at the centre of your practice. PCC is about the person, not their label.
- A person with LD might find it difficult to express their wishes, so be prepared to work with their family and carers too.
- If a person with LD can't make decisions for themself then you might have to be part of a 'best interests' process.   see *Section 6.1*

Notes

Capacity, consent and safeguarding

6.1 Mental capacity

How you work with people in your care is governed by several important legal frameworks, one of which is the **Mental Capacity Act (MCA) (2005)**.

Five key principles of the MCA (2005)

1. As LD nurses **we must assume that all people are able to make their own decisions**, unless it can be shown that they cannot do this.
2. **Provide as much support as you and the service can for people to make these decisions**. This would include all reasonable steps to help the individual to arrive at their own decisions. Example: use of assistive communication aids.
3. **Allowing people to make decisions that may appear unwise**. We must allow people the expression of their autonomy, even when this may seem an unwise action for them to do so. Example: consuming a great deal of alcohol.
4. **The concept of 'best interest'**. This is the idea that if people need decisions to be made on their behalf, then we should be able to demonstrate that these decisions are always taken with the *best interests* of the person concerned.
5. LD nurses and services should always seek the **least restrictive** way to enable people to lead a safe and full life.

Assessment of capacity

To consent to any form of care or treatment the person must have 'mental capacity'. If they lack mental capacity, they cannot give, or withhold consent.

See *Section 6.2* for more on consent

The use of DoLS (Deprivation of Liberty Safeguards)

This framework was originally introduced into the MCA in 2009 but is now in the process of being superseded by the introduction of the **Liberty Protection Safeguards (LPS)** legislation.

The DoLS were used to protect the rights of people who lack the ability (mental capacity) to make certain decisions for themselves and when it was necessary to deprive them of their liberty to keep them safe.

The two-question 'acid test' is used to see whether a person is being deprived of their liberty:

1. Is the person subject to continuous supervision and control? and
2. Is the person free to leave? – with the focus being not on whether a person seems to be wanting to leave, but on how those who support them would react if they did want to leave.

Notes

_____

_____

_____

_____

The use of LPS (Liberty Protection Safeguards)

In May 2019, the Mental Capacity (Amendment) Act was enacted into law. It has replaced the DoLS with a new scheme known as the Liberty Protection Safeguards (LPS).

This new law seeks to protect the liberty of people who do not have the mental capacity to make decisions about their care, but only covers England and Wales. It sets out to simplify the DoLS system; **however, it's not expected to come into legislative force until 2022**.

Some key features of the LPS are:

• One scheme will apply in all settings wherever people with LD live.
• It applies to anyone over the age of 16.
• The 'acid test' will be considered in relation to depriving a person of their liberty.

6.2 Consent

Whenever we work with people and do something to them, it's important we get consent for whatever it is.

Different types of consent are used in different circumstances.

The main types of consent are informal and formal, and it's important to gain the right type for whatever it is you're asking about. For example, if we are assisting a person to get dressed it'll soon get tedious if we ask for their permission in writing every time! In that situation, informal consent is appropriate, and a verbal 'yes' is perfectly adequate. People can also give informal implied consent. For example, if you ask a person if you can help them put on their shoes and they raise their foot, this could be considered implied consent; their actions demonstrate they are happy for you to go ahead.

However, you may be supporting someone who needs surgery or some other type of intervention. In this situation it's vital we gain formal consent, and the fact that the person has an LD does not mean that consent is not required.

In this situation it's important we consider the person's capacity to understand the information being given so they truly know what they are consenting (or not) to. Particularly with something such as surgery, there may be a lot of jargon and complicated language, so you may have to help them understand some of this. It may be appropriate that they have an advocate to support them. People with LD are susceptible to yielding to suggestions from the person asking questions, so an advocate can ensure this doesn't happen.

6.3 Safeguarding

Working with people with LD means that you will be working with some of the most vulnerable people in society. Safeguarding will be an important theme throughout your training and future career.

LD nurses are in a vital position to observe for types of abuse including:

- physical
- psychological
- neglect
- sexual
- financial
- discriminatory
- institutional.

Who should you report concerns to?

- If you suspect abuse, make sure that the immediate situation is safe; for example, is there a need for medical or police involvement?

- Report the disclosure to your practice assessor and university tutor without delay.
- Record all details, as you will need to be supported to make a written statement. This can be challenging but remember why courage is one of the 6 Cs!
- If someone discloses something you should listen and be sympathetic, but do not be judgemental or make any promises that you might not be able to keep.

If you have concerns about reporting to your practice assessor or university tutor, you can also report to a **Freedom to Speak up Guardian**. Guardians are employed by organisations as a confidential route to report safeguarding concerns. Their role is to channel the report to the most appropriate person to investigate.

Notes

_____

_____

_____

_____

_____

_____

_____

_____

Your social media accounts should be set to private. Don't befriend patients, relatives or practice colleagues. Remember they may be able to see some aspects of your profile even if you've used the security settings, so be mindful about profile pictures, etc.

There can be benefits to engaging with social media as a student. There are national groups, such as @WeLDnurses on Twitter, which provides a forum to engage with each other and reflect our professional identity (other groups are also available).

> Familiarise yourself with the NMC guidance on using social media, available at bit.ly/NMC-SM

Notes

Settling there

Make sure you've done your research and are familiar with the patient demographics and type of care delivered in your placement area. You should be given an orientation to the placement area on your first day, so find out if you need access codes/smart cards; where fire exits and assembly points are, the location of staff rooms, etc. It's also useful to find out the arrangements for handovers, e.g. time and locations, and what the local arrangements are for taking breaks/lunch.

Find out who to report to: who will your practice assessor and practice supervisor(s) be? If you're working in an area where there are no registered nurses then special arrangements will be in place; pay close attention to these and be sure to ask questions if you're unsure. Arrange your placement interviews and inform your academic assessor who your practice assessor is and give their contact details – be sure to follow local policy.

Try to establish your shifts/working hours early, as this will help you and your placement area to plan learning opportunities; try to be as flexible as possible. If you're on placement with other students try to ensure that you're not all on duty together as this can be overwhelming for staff and patients, as well as limiting the learning opportunities available to you all.

Notes

Working with those supervising your practice

Starting a new placement can be daunting; it can feel like starting a new job! Remember that the nurses you'll be working alongside will have been in the same position when they were students. You may find it useful to talk to more experienced students to find out how they settle into a new placement.

Whilst on placement you'll need to be prepared to ask questions. Don't be afraid to say that you don't know or are unsure about something. Discuss with your practice supervisor when the right time to ask questions will be; sometimes it's appropriate to ask questions right away, in other situations it may be better to note down your questions so they can be discussed later.

When you start your placement make sure that you've prepared a list of questions for your practice supervisor. This will ensure that you have the information you need to get the most out of your placement.

Your questions may include:

- working/shift patterns of your placement area
- how you will be supervised in practice and by whom
- who the other members of the team are and their roles
- opportunities for any insight visits
- their expectations for your role.

Whilst each placement area will have different documentation, you'll still see some common themes. These documents may be in paper or electronic form or both. You might also see some of the documents written in two formats – standard and easy read, so they are more accessible for people with LD. Some of the key documents are outlined below, with space for you to add any others you encounter.

Care plans	These highlight a need that an individual has and set out a detailed plan of how those supporting the person can meet that need in line with their wishes.
Health action plans (HAP)	HAPs are a larger collection of care plan documents that are written in an accessible format to support people with LD to manage their own health and wellbeing.
Hospital passports	Sometimes called traffic light documents because of their use of red, amber and green sections, these give an overview of what hospital staff need to know when caring for the individual.
Medication administration records	Dates, times, doses, routes and the names of each medication a person is prescribed will be detailed on this legal document. Nurses must sign this document every time they administer a medication.

One-page profiles	Often the most useful documents when starting a new placement, these are a snapshot of important information you need to know about an individual.
Risk assessments	These documents detail the likelihood that an adverse event will occur and if it does, the likely impact of this occurrence. They will also list the control measures that will reduce the chances of an adverse event.

Communicating with people with LD

Many people with LD will experience communication difficulties and it's important we take the time to find out how they communicate. Whilst we can look at their records and histories, there is no real shortcut to spending time with the person and their carers. Previous information is a useful way to gain insight but you should always check that the information is current and accurate, as individuals develop and change throughout the lifespan.

Augmentative and alternative communication

Augmentative and alternative communication (AAC) is the term used to identify any method of communication that supplements the 'normal' channels of communication. These strategies range in terms of complexity and cost. Whatever strategy you use, remember that the aim is to empower the person by allowing them to communicate their needs and wishes.

Objects of reference	These are items that are used to represent an item, person or activity. Connections can be learnt between the object and an activity, e.g. by providing a person with the object immediately before the activity.
Picture Exchange Communication System (PECS)	This system is used frequently with children. The child learns to associate pictures with objects or places that can be developed into a collection in a folder. The pictures can then be used to identify choices, e.g. food.

Makaton	Makaton is a form of sign language that is used in both child and adult settings. People do need functional vision and a level of manual dexterity to use Makaton and will often invent their own signs.
Multisensory	Multisensory rooms/environments provide valuable opportunities to test functional vision and hearing. The results of these assessments can then be used to plan communication strategies.
Voice output communication aids	These aids use technology to produce speech for people who have limited or no vocal output. There are many systems in use that include keyboard, head control and eyes to select words, to generate a voice output.

Accessible information

The accessible information standard set out by the UK Government in 2016 aimed to improve communication with people with disabilities through the following steps:

- Find out communication and information needs
- Record these needs clearly and consistently
- Flag these needs
- Share information and communication needs when required
- Take action to give the right support, e.g. offering accessible information.

LD nurses have an important role in educating other health and social care workers in providing information in accessible formats.

Notes

Being there

12.1 Hand hygiene

Hand washing is the best intervention that healthcare professionals can complete to help prevent the spread of healthcare-associated infections.

RUB HANDS FOR HAND HYGIENE! WASH HANDS WHEN VISIBLY SOILED

🕐 **Duartion of the entire procedure:** 20–30 seconds

Apply a palmful of the product in a cupped hand, covering all surfaces;

Rub hands palm to palm;

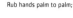

Right palm over left dorsum with interlaced fingers and vice versa;

Palm to palm with fingers interlaced;

Backs of fingers to opposing palms with fingers interlocked

Rotational rubbing of left thumb clasped in right palm and vice versa;

Rotational rubbing, backwards and forwards with clasped fingers of right hand in left palm and vice versa;

Once dry, your hands are safe.

Proper hand rub technique (World Health Organization, 2009). Reproduced with permission of the World Health Organization, www.who.int.

You're likely to have placements in community settings in addition to residential or hospital areas, and this might mean that you're not able to wash your hands with soap and water because the facilities aren't available. In situations where your hands are not soiled, you can use alcohol gel as an alternative; you can find a step-by-step guide to cleansing your hands on the opposite page.

12.2 Moving and handling

It's important when moving and handling to keep yourself safe as well as those you're supporting, so the first question to ask is 'do I need to move this person or object?'. If so, you can assess the risk using TILE.

Task	What do you want to do? What is the planned outcome of the task? e.g. assist the person out of bed.
Individual	What are your capabilities? Do you have any health conditions that might impact on your ability to perform the task safely?
Load	This refers to the person or object that you're moving. You might need some support or additional equipment, e.g. a hoist for a person who has PMLD.
Environment	Assess the area that you're working in and where you're moving the 'load' to – they must both be safe and free of any potential hazards.

 Notes

27

i Top tips

- For some people with PMLD the process of being moved can be disconcerting, so ensure you keep them informed of what is happening at each step.
- Each person you support will likely have different mobility needs and abilities, so make sure you're familiar with these before assisting them.
- If specialist equipment, such as hoists, is used to move people, you must ensure you're familiar with how to use it safely before carrying out the activity.
- Some people will have feeding tubes or other devices connected to them that might need to be moved safely with them.
- Think about your own body position when moving and handling; do not twist or lean.
- If a person looks like they are about to fall – do not catch them. This can be dangerous for them and you. Help them to the floor if it is safe to do so, then seek assistance.

✎ Notes

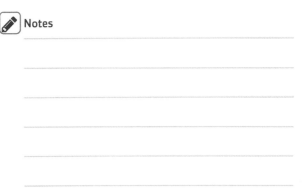

12.3 Challenging behaviour

On placement you may hear people or placement areas being described as having 'challenging behaviour'. In some services this is called different things and it may be referred to as 'behaviours of concern' or 'complex behaviours' but basically it means the same thing. In this book we will refer to it as challenging behaviour.

This may sound scary or intimidating so let's talk about what this means. There are several definitions of it but a seminal one is: "culturally abnormal behaviours of such intensity, frequency or duration that the physical safety of the person or others is placed in jeopardy, or behaviour that is likely to seriously limit or delay access to and use of ordinary community facilities" (Emerson *et al.*, 1987).

Breaking this definition down, we can see it talks about behaviours that are culturally abnormal; this can mean things such as inappropriate behaviours or antisocial behaviours. It also mentions 'intensity, frequency and duration' of the behaviour. This means that what we describe as a challenging behaviour may vary depending on these factors. For example, if a person screams once it may not be pleasant, but it's OK; however, if the person screams constantly all day that becomes problematic. So, the frequency and duration of that behaviour are determining that it is a challenge.

It also states behaviours that put the 'physical safety of the person or others in jeopardy' so this means either self-harming behaviours or violence and aggression towards other people. Finally, this definition says that challenging behaviour is any behaviour that stops people having 'access to and use

Emerson, E., Toogood, A., Mansell, J. et al. (1987) Challenging Behaviour and Community Services: 1. Introduction and overview. *Journal of the British Institute of Mental Handicap (APEX)*, 15(4): 166–169. Available at: bit.ly/S12-3.

of ordinary community facilities' – so that can be a whole range of antisocial and inappropriate behaviours.

When we use the term 'challenging behaviour' it's a huge phrase that can mean violence and aggression to others, self-harm/injury, destruction of property and/or socially unacceptable behaviours.

As a student you may be advised by the staff on placement to remove yourself from the area if a person is displaying challenging behaviours. Do not feel this is a bad thing or a reflection on you and your skills. It can make a difference to a situation when we know the person, knowing the right things to say, and the things not to say, so this will be why you're being advised to leave the area.

See *Section 13.4* for how we can support people who display challenging behaviours

Notes

13.1 Assessment

Assessment in nursing is the process by which the needs and abilities of an individual are identified through a structured process. It's important to establish what is usual for each person, so you have a basis for comparison.

Two common assessments that you might see in LD placements are discussed below.

Activities of daily living (ADL)

The ADL assessment was developed by Roper, Logan and Tierney and uses twelve activities of daily living to ensure a thorough and holistic assessment. The ADLs are listed below, along with a sample question to consider; there is then space to add your own.

1. Maintaining a safe environment
Is the environment clean and free of danger?

....

....

2. Communication
In what ways does the person wish to communicate?

....

....

3. Breathing

Does the person have any issues or conditions that might impact their breathing?

....

....

4. Eating and drinking

Do you have concerns about weight or fluid or nutritional intake?

....

....

5. Elimination

Is this person at risk of constipation?

see *Section 13.3*

....

....

6. Washing and dressing

Can the person manage this task independently or do they need support?

....

....

7. Controlling temperature

Are they feeling hot, cold, sweating or shivering?

....

....

8. **Mobilisation**
   Does the person need any assistance with mobilising?

   ....

   ....

9. **Working and playing**
   Work or day activities provide a meaningful sense of
   purpose; does this person have something they consider
   meaningful to do with their time?

   ....

   ....

10. **Expressing sexuality**
    Does the person know how to express their sexuality
    safely?

    ....

    ....

11. **Sleeping**
    Does the person have a usual and stable sleep pattern?

    ....

    ....

12. **Death and dying**
    If the person is being cared for by elderly parents, has
    any consideration been made as to what will happen to
    the person when their parents die?

    ....

    ....

Health Equality Framework (HEF)

The HEF is an evidence-based systemic measure developed by LD nurses and is part of the Moulster and Griffiths LD nursing model (see *Section 5*). It focuses on evidence of health inequalities experienced by people with LD across five broad categories (called 'determinants'):

- Social
- Genetic and biological
- Communication and health literacy
- Personal health behaviour and lifestyle risks
- Deficiencies in access to, and quality of, health provision.

Within these five determinants are indicators of health inequalities that a person with LD might experience. There are 29 health inequality indicators, each with their own unique descriptors to help you assess their impact. A score of 0–4 is given for every health inequality indicator; the greater the number, the greater the negative impact the indicator has on the life of the person.

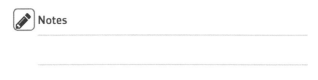

For a complete guide to the HEF and more information on the five determinants and individual descriptors go to: bit.ly/HEF-GP

Different placement areas will use different assessments and many will have developed their own to suit that service. Assessments will not solely focus on what a person cannot do but will highlight what a person can do for themselves.

Notes

Top tips

- Be mindful that sometimes people with LD will say what they think you want to hear.
- Don't forget to speak to a person's family, carers and staff to build a more thorough picture.
- Observation can also be a powerful assessment tool; spend time getting to know people. This also makes it easier for you to see when something might have changed.
- Not all assessments will be designed to be holistic; however, we always need to be open to additional factors that can influence these assessments.

13.2 Care planning

Care planning is a problem-solving cyclical approach that nurses use to deliver nursing care. It's often called the nursing process and consists of:

Assessment	Data collection; sources may include:
	• the person • carers • observations • assessment tools • old records • paramedics
	Skills required by the nurse include:
	• listening • observation • verbal/non-verbal communication • physical examination
Diagnosis	The nurse uses clinical judgement to identify nursing needs from the assessment data, resulting in clearly identified actual and potential nursing problems

Planning	Identification of goals and nursing interventions required to meet these goals. Goals should be SMART:
	• **S**pecific
	• **M**easurable
	• **A**chievable
	• **R**ealistic
	• **T**ime-limited
	Nursing interventions are practical tasks that will be undertaken and should be:
	• realistic
	• explicit
	• evidence-based
	• prioritised
	• involved (involve the person, carers and MDT)
	• goal-centred
Implementation	The delivery of the planned interventions, ensuring that the care delivered is recorded
Evaluation	Reviewing the goals to see if they have been achieved
	If not achieved, then reviewing the original assessment, goals and interventions
	This is where the process becomes cyclical, as you may return to the planning stage

Find out how this framework is implemented in your practice area. For example, is a model of nursing being used? Examples include those by Moulster and Griffiths (see *Section 5*), Orem (1980), Neuman (2011) and Roy (1980). These nursing models all have different philosophies as to how to approach the delivery of nursing care, but will adopt the principles of care planning.

Orem, D. (1980) *Nursing: concepts of practice.* McGraw-Hill.

Neuman, B. and Fawcett, J. (2011) *The Neuman Systems Model* (5th ed.). Pearson.

Roy, C. (1980) *Introduction to Nursing: an adaptation model.* Prentice Hall.

13.3 Constipation management

People with LD are more at risk of constipation than the general population. Constipation can be caused by poor fluid or fibre intake, limited physical activity or medication side-effects. Constipation is preventable and treatable, but sadly people with LD have died due to complications from severe constipation. The cycle below looks at how this can happen.

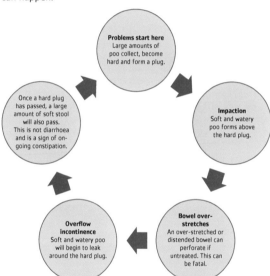

The constipation cycle. Based on information from NHS England's 'Poo matters' campaign and licensed for use via the Open Government Licence.

It's important to know when action needs to be taken with constipation, therefore you might be involved in monitoring the bowel output of an individual. The most common chart referred to in this process is the Bristol Stool Chart.

> A copy of the Bristol Stool Chart is
> provided on the inside back cover

Type 4 and 5 stools are healthy but if you notice that a person is consistently passing stools outside of this range it may be a sign that they're constipated, and you should escalate your findings.

13.4 Managing challenging behaviour

Many services use an approach called positive behaviour support (PBS). It's aimed at understanding why the person displays challenging behaviours and how we can support them to reduce those behaviours. It should include detailed assessments to understand the behaviour, then developing a plan that involves proactive strategies (to avoid the behaviour occurring) and reactive strategies (how we can support the person when the behaviours do occur). PBS should focus on improving the quality of life for the person, it should be person-centred and non-punitive.

PBS is an excellent approach but there will be times where it does not work or has not been implemented yet, such as if the person is new to the placement. In these situations, you may be encouraged to use de-escalation approaches. De-escalation is aimed at reducing the incident through calm approaches; think about your body language, what you say, how you say it and – most importantly – listen to the person. If you've not been trained in this, you should leave it to the placement staff.

Some services may also use physical intervention techniques. There are many different types of physical interventions and it's vital you do not get involved with these unless trained in the correct one for your placement whilst you're there.

Some placement areas use personal safety alarms. Where this is the case it's vital you use the alarm as advised by the placement staff following their local procedures.

When you work with people who display challenging behaviour it's important to remember that people do not *have* challenging behaviour in the same way a person has a cold or measles; people *display* challenging behaviour and this will be a result of something else, a reaction to their circumstances; challenging behaviour may be a means of getting their message across.

13.5 Medication management

On placement you may be involved in medication management; this may mean drug administration or supporting a person to self-medicate.

When involved in this it's important to remember the 9 rights:

1. Right **patient/person**
2. Right **medication**
3. Right **dose**
4. Right **time**
5. Right **route**
6. Right **reason**
7. Right **documentation**
8. Right **patient education**
9. Right **response**

Some literature also talks about a tenth right, the right to refuse.

Medication errors can happen. As a student you're not allowed to administer medication alone, but you should understand the importance of doing the right thing if an error occurs. All nurses have a duty of candour, which means we must be open and honest with patients when something goes wrong with their treatment or care. This means we must report it as soon as possible. It will be vital that the person who made the error is supported and that the person with LD is closely monitored for any adverse effects and supported too.

There has been criticism in recent years about the use of medication to control challenging behaviours when there is no diagnosis of mental ill health. This has led to a national project called 'Stopping the over-medication of people with a learning disability' referred to as STOMP. STOMP (2018) claim that people with LD, autism or both are being prescribed antipsychotic medication, an antidepressant, or both, without the appropriate diagnosis for such, which can lead to many severe side-effects including organ failure and death. It's useful to be aware of this and staff should be looking to reduce the use of these types of medication.

> You can find out more about STOMP at: bit.ly/STO-MP

13.6 Mental health

People living with LD may express their emotional distress and experiences in different ways compared to the general population.

Some common mental health conditions you'll encounter are shown below.

Anxiety

Anxiety is the body's natural protective response when encountering a threat. It involves the body mobilising its resources to 'fight, flight or freeze'. For people with LD this can be communicated by:

- excessive pacing
- an increase in general agitated behaviour
- an increase in self-harming behaviour or towards objects within their environment
- an increase, or reduction, in their verbal expression and behaviour, including a change in the language that you wouldn't normally associate with them.

Depression

This relates to how a person reflects upon, thinks and feels about their mood. For people with LD this can be communicated by:

- excessive pacing
- an increase in agitated behaviour
- becoming more withdrawn and quieter than is usual for them
- an increase in self-harm
- eating much more, or a sudden loss of appetite
- an increase or reduction in their verbal expression and behaviour
- a change in their usual sleeping pattern.

Dementia

This refers to some organic deterioration in the brain that can affect an individual in several ways. It principally affects their cognitive abilities, which means the person may struggle in the areas of memory, language or the ability to undertake previous behaviours and activities that you would usually expect them to perform, e.g. washing or dressing themselves.

As you can see from the non-exhaustive list above, there is often an overlap and commonalities in possible behaviours that might occur, and recognising changes in behaviour is strongly associated with knowing the person well.

✏ Notes

41

13.7 Observations

The assessment of basic physical observations is used as an indicator as to whether the person's condition is improving or declining, and can be an early warning indicator of a life-threatening decline.

> See *Section 19* for normal observation ranges

Respiration rate:

- Count for one minute how many breaths the person takes.

Oxygen saturation level:

- Peripheral oxygen saturation (SpO_2) measures the amount of oxygen-carrying haemoglobin in the blood and the reading is usually taken using a pulse oximeter.
- It's important to note if the patient is on any supplementary oxygen as this will impact the reading.

Blood pressure:

- Use the right size cuff on your patient – very large or very small arms may need a non-standard size.
- Blood pressure readings can vary from minute to minute and can be influenced by a range of factors including pain, temperature, hydration, anxiety and body position.
- If you get a reading that you're concerned about, check the other arm as a comparison.

Heart rate:

- This is usually checked with a machine; however, it can also be done manually. If you're feeling for a pulse manually, remember not to use your thumb as you might be feeling your own pulse by mistake.
- Checking a pulse manually will also allow you to feel for strength and rhythm.

Temperature:

• Body temperature can vary from person to person, but the normal range is usually between 36°C and 37.5°C.

> **Remember:** if any vital signs are not within the normal ranges or you're concerned for any reason, it's vital that you inform the nurse and/or the responsible person working with you

Top tips

- If you're unsure how to take an observation reading, then you must ask your practice supervisor, as readings must be accurate.
- You will often take observations using machines; however, manual readings can also be taken and are a good way to check if you have an abnormal reading.
- Be mindful that people with LD might find the process of having their observations taken distressing.
- It's important to have a baseline for observations when the person is well, so that you know what is usual for them. This means you'll be able to spot any changes quickly.
- Informal observations are also important and can inform this more formal procedure. For example, you might notice a change in behaviour which might prompt you to check physical observations.

13.8 Palliative care
Learning Disabilities Mortality Review (LeDeR)

People with LD are three times more likely than the general population to die from conditions that could be treated. The average life expectancy of a person with LD is 19.7 years lower than the general population.

The LeDeR study aims to:

- support improvements in the quality of health and social care services for people with LD
- reduce premature mortality and health inequalities for people with LD.

Palliative care

Palliative care aims to improve the quality of life for people and their carers faced with life-threatening illness. Pain management is a key part of palliative care, but it encompasses far more than this, assessing and managing the physical, psychosocial and spiritual needs of the individual.

Being involved in palliative and end of life care

Caring for someone towards and at the end of their life is a unique and privileged role. Nurses can promote and provide quality care and support to fulfil the wishes and needs of the individual and their carers at the end of life's journey. This support may continue with the individual and carers after death.

Every individual and their carers have the right to request that students do not participate in their care. It's not unexpected that at this most intimate of moments many people express the desire to be with staff who they may have got to know over a prolonged period. Please do not be offended if you're not involved in certain aspects of the care required pre- and post-death, as people's wishes must be respected.

If you're involved in end of life care, it's recommended that you debrief with your practice assessor and staff on shift as soon as practicably possible. This has been proven to be effective in allowing students to process events and to enhance their confidence and skills for future practice.

13.9 People with autism

While on placement you will work with people with autism. Autism is often referred to as the autistic spectrum disorder or the autistic spectrum condition. The reason it's referred to in this way is because the way in which autism manifests and how it impacts on the person vary enormously. Some people with autism can have severe LD and high levels of need; others will be highly intelligent people who live ordinary lives; and others will come somewhere in between these two ends of the spectrum.

If you work with people with autism, like anyone else, it's vital you work in a person-centred way and there is not 'one way' you should work with people with autism. However, there are some key factors to bear in mind. Many people with autism have sensory impairments which can mean that the way their brain processes sensory information is different to yours, and this can cause challenges to them.

The second thing to consider is the way you communicate. Take care to think about what you say, and avoid 'sayings' or phrases that can be misinterpreted. For example, avoid saying 'in a minute' as the person may expect you to be there in literally 60 seconds.

13.10 Reasonable adjustments

The Equality Act (2010) places a legal duty on services, including health and social care providers, to make changes so their services are just as accessible to people with disabilities as they are for the general population. The Act calls these changes reasonable adjustments.

People with LD will sometimes face barriers when they try to access services. In these cases, your role might be advocating on behalf of the person with LD when they need reasonable adjustments making.

There is often confusion about the difference between equality and equity. People with LD need access to equitable services. What this means is shown in the cartoon below.

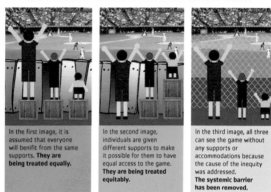

In the first image, it is assumed that everyone will benifit from the same supports. **They are being treated equally.**

In the second image, individuals are given different supports to make it possible for them to have equal access to the game. **They are being treated equitably.**

In the third image, all three can see the game without any supports or accommodations because the cause of the inequity was addressed. **The systemic barrier has been removed.**

A cartoon illustrating equality versus equity. Reproduced courtesy of Advancing Equity and Inclusion by City for All Women Initiative (CAWI), Ottawa.

The ultimate goal is to remove all potential barriers.

Below are some examples of common barriers that people with LD face when accessing services, with some suggested reasonable adjustments to overcome them. There is space for you to make notes on any additional barriers you might encounter when supporting individuals.

Barrier	Suggestions to overcome
Understanding People with LD can struggle to understand new and complicated information.	Offer a relative or carer the chance to attend the appointment, provide information in alternative formats, think creatively – can the information be explained another way using an analogy or objects of reference?

Barrier	Suggestions to overcome
Communication This can be a barrier for both people with LD and the staff who are working with them. Knowing the best way to communicate with a person can take time.	Communication passports, information from family and reviewing information from past appointments can all aid communication. However, there is no substitute for taking the time to get to know a person and using active and effective listening to find out from them the way they prefer to communicate.
Attitudes of staff/ services You may find that you're working with staff who do not understand the complexities of LD.	Staff may need basic LD awareness information. It's likely they are being cautious so as not to offend or upset the person with LD, therefore you can role model good practice for them.

- If you notice some barriers within your placement area you might feel awkward about addressing these yourself – if this is the case speak to your practice supervisor and discuss what you've noticed.
- Sometimes services can be reluctant to adopt reasonable adjustments, as they can be seen as time- and/or resource-intensive. It's useful to remember that time invested now can save significant resources in the long term, as reasonable adjustments can be useful for everyone who accesses a service, not just people with LD.

13.11 Risk assessments

Risk assessment is one aspect of overall risk management strategies within a practice area and addresses the following questions:

- How likely is the event to occur?
- How soon is it expected to occur?
- How severe will the outcome be?

Risk factors

- Static factors – these are unchangeable, e.g. a person's history
- Dynamic factors – these are changeable, e.g. drug and alcohol use
- Chronic factors – these are slow-changing dynamic factors
- Acute factors/triggers, rapidly changing factors.

Different practice areas may use different risk assessment tools so check with your practice supervisor to find out what specific tools are used in your placement area.

Positive risk taking

Taking risks is an important aspect of personal development and we all need to take risks and learn from mistakes. If you consider normal child development, at some point safety factors are relaxed for development to take place; this might be walking to school alone, making a hot drink, etc.

Equally, people with an LD, to be able to live socially normative lives, must be supported to take risks. Not to allow this could result in risk avoidance, sometimes called being risk averse.

It's important that when engaging in positive risk taking in practice, risk assessments are completed and that the activity is overseen by the MDT.

Lone working

There will be times when you'll engage in lone working; for example, community visits or escorting. Lone working may mean that the ability to have close support from other staff or to withdraw from a situation is restricted or limited.

Each organisation must have a lone worker policy and is responsible for carrying out risk assessments to manage the risk to lone workers, reducing the risk of harm.

13.12 Working with children

You're most likely to encounter children or young people with LD in an educational or respite care setting. There are also peripatetic services that support families, such as child and adolescent mental health services (CAMHS) and specialist community nurses.

Education

In education (special needs nursery, school, further education college) you will need to become familiar with the daily activities, routines and roles of the multi-professional team.

You will have the opportunity to work with the teaching staff, speech therapists, occupational therapists, physiotherapists, and possibly educational psychologists and parents. Each child will have an Education, Health and Care Plan which details the care and support they need.

Sometimes there will be a nurse working on site with you; their focus is on providing care for children with complex healthcare needs.

Respite care

Respite care settings for children with LD provide 24-hour care in a home-from-home setting. This enables parents and families to take a break and may be for a single night or up to a few weeks.

CAMHS

LD teams within CAMHS support children with an LD and additional emotional, mental health or behavioural needs. Their role is to work with the family to assess children and identify interventions and support strategies. You might be involved in supporting clinics, outreach services or crisis intervention.

Specialist community nurse

The specialist community nurse works closely with parents or carers, focusing on healthcare issues such as toilet training and continence, eating and drinking, behaviour, constipation, dental care and sleep.

Top tips

- Do not talk over the child – always involve them in discussions
- Promote choice
- Allow extra time for a response
- Use communication aids
- Kneel to talk to small children
- Talk to the child in an age-appropriate way
- Ensure that the child is in a safe and comfortable position for eating, drinking, sleeping, learning and playing
- Always use play! This is helpful for assessment, communication, teaching and building a relationship.

Transition

The transition from child to adult can be a confusing and challenging time.

Some families have described reaching adulthood as if they were on a 'cliff edge' where all support is withdrawn, with no adult equivalent available. To avoid this, the transition from child to adult services is carefully planned in partnership with the young person and their family. Starting the process early can help to minimise anxiety, promote consistency in care and provide a gradual and seamless transition.

 Notes

Basic Life Support (BLS) is something that all student nurses/ nurses are trained to undertake if a patient has either a respiratory or cardiac arrest. These are emergency situations that will usually require specialist healthcare interventions, so at the outset it's important to recognise that your role is to spot the situation, call for help and initiate BLS, as outlined below.

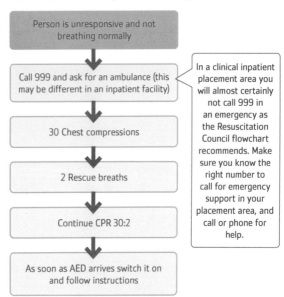

Person is unresponsive and not breathing normally

Call 999 and ask for an ambulance (this may be different in an inpatient facility)

In a clinical inpatient placement area you will almost certainly not call 999 in an emergency as the Resuscitation Council flowchart recommends. Make sure you know the right number to call for emergency support in your placement area, and call or phone for help.

30 Chest compressions

2 Rescue breaths

Continue CPR 30:2

As soon as AED arrives switch it on and follow instructions

Adult Basic Life Support (Resuscitation Council, 2015).
CPR 30:2 – an emergency cardiopulmonary resuscitation procedure that alternates 30 chest compressions with two rescue breaths; AED – automated external defibrillator (a portable device that checks the heart rhythm and can send an electric shock to the heart to try to restore a normal rhythm). Reproduced with the kind permission of the Resuscitation Council (UK).

Do not attempt resuscitation (DNAR) orders

For some, the decision may be made that if they were to have an arrest they should be allowed to die peacefully. If this decision is to be made, the person and their carers should be involved in the decision-making process and the writing of a DNAR order. As a student nurse/nurse you should check the resuscitation status of service users. Unless you're certain that a current DNAR is in place, you must assume that the person is for resuscitation.

Complication of physical disabilities

Many people with an LD will have associated physical disabilities, which may for example change their chest shape. If this is the case the nurse should plan on an individual basis how to manage an arrest in the event of the situation arising. Individuals may have complex resuscitation plans, including manual handling, so make sure that you familiarise yourself with these when on placement.

Notes

15.1 Epilepsy

Epilepsy is a neurological condition categorised by recurrent seizures; one in three people with an LD also has some form of epilepsy, and it is more prominent in people with severe LD. People with an LD can show behaviour which may not be related to epilepsy; therefore, seizures may go unrecognised.

Broad signs and symptoms of epilepsy include:

- temporary confusion
- a staring spell
- uncontrollable jerking movements of the arms and legs
- loss of consciousness or awareness
- fear, anxiety or déjà vu.

Seizures are broadly categorised into two types: focal (affecting one part of the brain) and generalised (affecting both sides of the brain).

The presentation of a focal seizure depends on the part of the brain affected.

The different types of generalised seizures are:

- absence
- tonic–clonic or convulsive
- atonic (also known as drop attacks)
- clonic
- tonic
- myoclonic.

The type of seizure most people will think of is the convulsive generalised tonic–clonic. They can be frightening to watch, and someone who has one rarely knows or remembers what happened.

1 **For someone having a generalised tonic–clonic seizure**

- Make note of the time (this is one reason why a nurse always has a watch)
- Give them room – keep other people back
- Clear hard or sharp objects, like spectacles and furniture, away
- Cushion their head
- Loosen clothing around their neck if you can safely do so
- Don't hold them or stop their movements
- Don't put anything in their mouth
- Speak calmly, reassure them
- Stay until they're fully aware of where they are and can respond normally when you talk to them
- Don't give them anything to drink or eat until they've completely recovered.

Epilepsy can be treated through multiple strategies. Commonly, medication is needed to control seizures; these commonly prescribed drugs are called anticonvulsants. Other forms of treatment can be a procedure that removes or alters an area of the brain where seizures originate, vagus nerve stimulation (VNS – a procedure to put a small electrical device inside the body) and a ketogenic diet.

1 **When to seek emergency help**

- It's a person's first seizure
- The seizure lasts longer than 5 minutes
- Another seizure begins soon after the first
- The person doesn't 'wake up' after the movements have stopped
- The person was injured during the seizure.

15.2 Sepsis

There are 147 000 cases of sepsis per year in England and around 37 000 associated deaths. NHS England commissioned a national focus on sepsis in people with an LD, to raise awareness about prevention, identification and early treatment.

Sepsis is a time-critical medical emergency, which can occur as part of the body's immune system overreaction response to infection or injury.

With early diagnosis, sepsis can be treated with antibiotics. If not treated immediately, sepsis can result in organ failure and death.

Spotting sepsis in adults

- Slurred speech or confusion
- Extreme shivering or muscle pain
- Passing no urine (in a day)
- Severe breathlessness
- It feels like you're going to die
- Skin mottled or discoloured.

Spotting sepsis in children

- If the child is unwell with either a fever or very low temperature (or has had a fever in the last 24 hours)
- Is breathing very fast
- Has a 'fit' or convulsion
- Looks mottled, bluish, or pale
- Has a rash that doesn't fade when you press it
- Is very lethargic or difficult to wake
- Feels abnormally cold to touch.

A child under 5 may have sepsis if:

- they're not feeding
- they're vomiting repeatedly
- they haven't passed urine for 12 hours

> **If you suspect sepsis inform your practice colleagues immediately**

15.3 Choking

Approximately one in three people with LD will have some swallowing difficulties (also known as dysphagia); this means that they are more at risk of choking than the general population. Choking occurs when a foreign object (which can be something edible or inedible) gets stuck in the back of the throat and causes a blockage.

Blockages can be mild or severe.

Blockage type	Presentation	Treatment
Mild	People are usually unable to speak, cough, cry or breathe properly Individuals can usually clear mild blockages themselves with an adequate coughing reflex; however, this is not always the case	1. Ask the person if they are choking; if they can speak and cough, they can clear their own throat 2. Encourage the person to continue coughing
Severe	A severe blockage will mean that a person cannot cough, speak, cry or breathe and without support they will eventually become unconscious and collapse	1. Give up to five back blows 2. Give up to five abdominal thrusts 3. Check their mouth for any obvious signs of obstruction 4. If the obstruction does not clear after steps 1 and 2, call the emergency services/ for emergency help and repeat the process until help arrives

Be careful of your own safety – first aid guidance will sometimes recommend you remove any obvious obstructions from the person's mouth if you can see them. A person with LD and/or physical disabilities may not have the ability to control their jaw movement, particularly when they are distressed in a choking situation. It's important that you do not put yourself at risk – instead, call for emergency assistance.

People with PMLD are more likely to be at risk from choking and are more likely to have additional physical disabilities that can make back blows and/or abdominal thrusts difficult to perform. If individuals in your placement area are at significant risk of choking, they will have a risk assessment with control measures specific to their needs and you should familiarise yourself with this.

15.4 Sending a person with LD to A&E

Contact A&E in advance to let them know that you're bringing a person with LD and of any reasonable adjustments which would support that person, such as a separate room to wait in, prioritisation and additional staff support.

What to take

- **Hospital passport**
  These are designed to give hospital staff useful information about the person to help support them whilst in hospital. This includes information ranging from a person's current medication to their likes/dislikes.
- **Current medication**
  Take a list of, and take with you, the person's current medication. Make sure you know when they should take their medication so it can be administered if needed.

- **Contact information for carers, next of kin**
  This should be in the person's hospital passport, but ensure you have this information easily accessible to you.
- **Eating and drinking plans**
  Does the person have specific eating and drinking needs? Make sure any plans are passed on to hospital staff.

Top tips

- **How does the person show they are in pain?**
  Consider how you would know if the person you're supporting is in pain.

  > For more about pain see *Section 16*

- **Physical examinations/procedures**
  How does the person tolerate procedures, for example having a blood test? It's important to be aware what has helped the person in the past, e.g. anaesthetic cream, distraction techniques, PRN medication, etc.
- **Communication**
  Prepare the person with an LD (as much as possible in an emergency) for going to hospital, as this could be their first time.

  > See *Section 11* for communication tips

- **LD Liaison Team**
  Have you contacted the Acute LD Liaison Team? They can:
  - ensure the person is flagged as having an LD on the hospital systems
  - support the ward with reasonable adjustments, including providing easy read information.

Discharge

The person may be discharged home after a visit to A&E, so ensure that all information has been communicated clearly to carers at home/the next staff on shift. Has the person got adequate support in place at home? Do alternative arrangements need to be made, e.g. increased support?

Be clear on the plan for aftercare, what signs and symptoms to look out for and when to escalate and seek further help. Also support the person with an LD to understand this.

📝 **Notes**

_____

_____

_____

_____

_____

_____

_____

_____

_____

_____

_____

Pain and pain assessment

The feeling of pain is a subjective experience, and research has shown that people with LD are less likely to receive pain relief than the general population. This may partly be because people with more severe LD might find it difficult to express when they are in pain and those working with them may find it difficult to notice non-verbal signs. Therefore, it's important for everyone to be aware when a person might be experiencing discomfort.

Here are some non-verbal signs for you to look out for that might indicate pain:

- Grimacing or face pulling
- Unusual facial expressions
- Crying or distressed vocalising
- Changes in behaviour
- Reduced activity and/or mobility
- Withdrawn
- Unusual reactions to touch.

Pain passports can be helpful to determine how a person with LD will usually present when they are pain-free and how this might compare to when they are experiencing pain.

DisDAT

Formerly called the Disability Distress Assessment Tool, the more recently renamed Distress and Discomfort Assessment Tool (DisDAT) is used to establish a baseline for individuals, describing how they present when they are content versus how they might present when they are distressed and/or in pain. This information can be used to compare signs, behaviours and observations that a person might be experiencing pain.

> For more information on the DisDAT and to find a copy of the latest version visit: bit.ly/disDAT

17 | Common groups of medications

As people with LD tend to have additional needs, you're likely to encounter a vast range of medications that are used to treat both physical and mental health conditions. Some common groups of medications are detailed in the table below, with space for you to note down others you may encounter.

Medication group	Reason for medication	Medication names (not an exhaustive list)
Analgesics	Pain relief	Paracetamol, ibuprofen, co-codamol, codeine, tramadol
Anti-arrhythmics	Irregular heartbeat	Digoxin
Antibiotics	Bacterial infection	Penicillins, erythromycin, clarithromycin, vancomycin, metronidazole
Anticoagulants	Blood thinner	Aspirin, rivaroxaban, heparin, warfarin
Anti-emetic	Nausea/ anti-sickness	Metoclopramide, ondansetron, cyclizine
Antihistamines	Control allergies	Cetirizine, cyclizine, chlorphenamine maleate
Antihypertensive	Lowers blood pressure	ACE inhibitors, beta-blockers, calcium channel blockers

Medication group	Reason for medication	Medication names (not an exhaustive list)
Anxiolytics	Anxiety	Diazepam, lorazepam, chlordiazepoxide
Diuretic	Water pill/fluid retention	Furosemide, bendroflumethiazide
Laxatives	Constipation	Docusate, senna, suppositories
Statins	Cholesterol-reducing	Simvastatin, atorvastatin, lovastatin

Notes

Notes

Moving on from there

Reflection is a process widely encouraged for student nurses and is required of you by the NMC for revalidation when you're qualified. Like many skills, though, reflection often takes practice and the more we do it, the better we get at it.

There are many models of reflection available and these are useful in helping us to develop those skills. The models can help guide the thought process and help us avoid getting bogged down in the negatives of a situation. The purpose of reflection is that we learn and develop, it's not a process to show ourselves how bad we are at something. We can acknowledge mistakes and errors but also look at positives and how we can improve next time.

There are many reflective models around, so it's useful to have a look and find the ones that work for you. Some are more suitable for certain situations than others.

The model below is useful for critical incident reflecting, so may suit situations that arise on placement.

The REFLECT Model (Barksby, Butcher and Whysall, 2015)

This model conveniently uses the word *reflect* as a mnemonic to help us remember each stage.

Barksby, J., Butcher, N. and Whysall, A. (2015) A new model of reflection for clinical practice. *Nursing Times*, 111: 34/35, 21–23.

	Explanation	Action
R	RECALL the events	A brief overview of the situation
E	EXAMINE our responses	Examine your thoughts and actions at the time
F	Acknowledge FEELINGS	Highlight your feelings at the time
L	LEARN from the experience	What have you learnt from the experience?
E	EXPLORE options	Discuss your options for the future
C	CREATE a plan of action	An action plan for the future
T	Set TIMESCALE	Set timescales by which the plan in the previous step will be completed

Other models that are commonly used in nursing include
Gibbs' (1988) and Johns' (1997) but many people like Borton's
(1970) model. This one has three stages and although often
regarded as a simple model, it nonetheless still covers the key
areas required for the reflective process and like REFLECT, is
very easy to remember.

Borton's model consists of:

- Stage 1: **What?**
- Stage 2: **So what?**
- Stage 3: **Now what?**

Have a go at using a variety of reflective models until you
decide which one you like best.

Borton, T. (1970) *Reach, Touch and Teach.* McGraw-Hill.

67

Definition of a learning disability

Below is the accepted Department of Health definition of an LD that comes from a 2001 Government White Paper, *Valuing People: a new strategy for learning disability for the 21st century.*

> You can read the paper in full at:
> bit.ly/S19-LD

Impaired intelligence
(a significantly reduced ability to understand new or complex information, to learn new skills)
...with...

Impaired social functioning
(a reduced ability to cope independently)
...which...

Started **before adulthood** with a **lasting effect on development**

Until version 11 of the International Classification of Diseases was published in 2018, an IQ of <70 was recognised as being an integral part of an LD diagnosis. However, this no longer forms part of the international definition of an LD, as relying on an IQ alone omits any measure of social or adaptive abilities.

Other terms used for learning disabilities

'Learning disability' is the primary term used within the UK; however, intellectual disability is also becoming more widespread. Some common terms for learning disabilities used globally are:

- Intellectual disability
- Developmental disability
- Intellectual developmental disorder
- Neurodevelopmental disorder.

Severity of LD

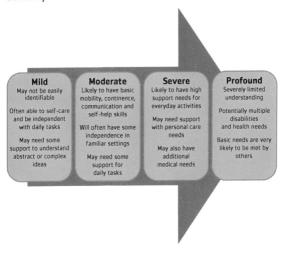

Mild
May not be easily identifiable

Often able to self-care and be independent with daily tasks

May need some support to understand abstract or complex ideas

Moderate
Likely to have basic mobility, continence, communication and self-help skills

Will often have some independence in familiar settings

May need some support for daily tasks

Severe
Likely to have high support needs for everyday activities

May need support with personal care needs

May also have additional medical needs

Profound
Severely limited understanding

Potentially multiple disabilities and health needs

Basic needs are very likely to be met by others

The difference between a learning disability and a learning difficulty

Learning disability and learning difficulty are two different terms but they tend to be used interchangeably in the media; however, they do not mean the same thing. A learning difficulty is not a significant general impairment of intelligence and tends to be used in UK education settings to refer to conditions such as dyslexia.

> The differences are explained by
> Mencap at bit.ly/Mencap-LD

Normal ranges for basic vital sign observations

Respiratory rate	12–20 breaths per minute
Oxygen saturation	94–99%
Blood pressure	100/60 – 140/80 mmHg
Heart/pulse rate	60–100 beats per minute
Temperature	36–37.5°C

Remember these are usual ranges for a healthy adult. People with LD who have additional comorbidities may have their own baseline for what is usual for them.

Metric units and their equivalents

Unit	Abbreviation	Equivalent	Abbreviation
1 kilogram	kg	1000 grams	g
1 gram	g	1000 milligrams	mg
1 milligram	mg	1000 micrograms	mcg*
1 microgram	mcg*	1000 nanograms	ng*
1 litre	L or l	1000 millilitres	ml
1 mole	mol	1000 millimoles	mmol
1 millimole	mmol	1000 micromoles	mcmol

*It's recommended that these units should not be abbreviated and should be written out in full to avoid potential misreading.

Infection control waste bags

Bin colour	Use	Examples of waste
Black	Domestic/general waste	Food waste
Yellow	Hazardous/infectious waste	Gloves, aprons, items with bodily fluids
Yellow with black line	Offensive waste	Soiled continence aids
Purple	Cytotoxic waste	Chemotherapy drugs
Orange	Infectious waste	Dressings

Notes

My placement does not have a registered nurse –
how will I meet my outcomes?

At the start of the placement discuss your planned
learning outcomes with your practice supervisor; they
will be able to guide you with realistic expectations
for your placement area. Placement areas without
registered nurses are great opportunities to focus
on the fundamentals of care, working alongside
other professionals and supporting people with
LD and their families by practising skills such as
communication, personal care and MDT working.

What do I do if I make a mistake in practice?

Don't panic, and be honest. Mistakes will happen,
especially when you're new to the profession. It's
important that you tell someone as soon as possible –
this is the standard that the NMC expects from qualified
nurses and it applies to students too. From there, a
plan can be devised on how to deal with the mistake,
depending on the severity of the issue.

What does it mean for me to have supernumerary
status?

Whilst on placement you should be a supernumerary
member of the team. This means you are in addition
to the other staff who already work in that area.
This allows you to focus on your learning and
gaining experience. If you feel you're not treated

as a supernumerary staff member, speak to either your practice supervisor or academic assessor.

What happens if I don't feel comfortable when being asked to do something in practice?

It's important to be open and honest about your skills and competence. Talk to your practice supervisor or the person you're working with and let them know how you feel. You should only perform tasks that you feel confident and competent to complete, so you should feel free to say that this is not the case. Use this as a learning opportunity and ask to observe whilst someone with the skill performs the task. This can help grow your knowledge, so next time, you may feel more able.

What happens if I don't like my practice supervisor and/or my placement?

Remember that placements are not forever. Try to make the most of any experience, organise insight days, work with other teams who interact with your placement and spend time getting to know the people you're supporting. Continue to stay positive, professional and respectful and try to make the most out of what you've experienced.

What do I do if I witness poor practice or have concerns about care?

It depends on the severity of the situation but in the first instance you should discuss it with the most senior person on duty or your practice supervisor. If you do not feel able to do this, then you should talk to your academic assessor. Remember that if you see poor care and have safeguarding concerns you have a duty of care to report this to someone senior.

British Institute of Learning Disabilities: www.bild.org.uk

Easy Health (for accessible information): www.easyhealth.org.uk

Easy on the i: www.easyonthei-leeds.nhs.uk

Health Education England: www.hee.nhs.uk/our-work/learning-disability

Learning Disability Practice: https://journals.rcni.com/learning-disability-practice

Learning Disability Today: www.learningdisabilitytoday.co.uk

Mencap: www.mencap.org.uk

Notes

_____

_____

_____

_____

_____

_____

_____

Notes

Notes

Notes

Notes